Snoozby and the Great Big Bedtime Battle

Terry Cralle

W. David Brown

Illustrated by Margeaux Lucas

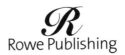

Rowe Publishing

SOFTCOVER
ISBN 13: 978-1-939054-38-8
ISBN 10: 1-939054-38-9

HARDCOVER
ISBN 13: 978-1-939054-47-0
ISBN 10: 1-939054-47-8

Illustrated by Margeaux Lucas.

3 5 7 9 8 6 4 2

Printed in the United States of America
Published by

R
Rowe Publishing

www.rowepub.com
Stockton, Kansas

This book is dedicated to

Genevieve Piturro

and The Pajama Program;

providing new pajamas and new books

to children in need nationwide,

and to our sleep superheroes

Den

David

Christopher

and

Will

http://www.pajamaprogram.org

Dear Friends, Parents and Educators,

Simply put, sufficient sleep is a win-win proposition. Sleep helps everyone think better, learn better, focus better—and just plain do better. Yet many adults fail to understand the importance of sleep health and wellness, let alone effectively communicate that message to children.

Sleep affects the quality of our lives in many ways. Our need for sleep is as basic as our need for food and water, and it must be considered as such if we are to lead healthy lives. Sleep, diet and exercise form the very foundation of health and well-being.

Meeting daily sleep requirements maximizes thinking, learning, memory, productivity, mood, decision-making, behavior, focus, judgment and safety for adults and children alike. It is imperative that children understand the importance of sufficient sleep if they are to reach their full potential. If we can help children understand why we all need sleep, as well as the importance and benefits of sufficient sleep, bedtime can easily become a positive, relaxing, peaceful and reflective time of day.

It is critical that we view sleep with positivity and respect. We urge adults to never use sleep or an early bedtime as a punishment or negative consequence for a child of any age. When everyone's knowledge and awareness about sleep is increased, sufficient sleep becomes a personal value as well as a family, community, and societal value.

As sleep educators and clinicians, we believe it is never too early to start the dialogue about sleep. Sleep research has demonstrated that getting sufficient, quality sleep is vitally important, especially for children. Therefore, it is essential to instill good sleep habits in our children to achieve the maximum benefits that healthy sleep provides, as well as to lay the foundation for a healthier and happier adulthood and enhanced quality of life.

Demonstrating that sleep is for winners and providing an overview of the daytime benefits of nighttime sleep are our goals for this book. In the first of the *Snoozby* sleep series, we provide the basic tenets of the benefits of quality sleep—based on current sleep-medicine research—in an easy-to-read format. Children's fundamental awareness and understanding of the value of sleep will lead to improved attitudes and responses from both children and parents to bedtime, to falling asleep, and to waking up during the night.

We encourage parents and educators to discuss sleep early and often with children in an effort to reinforce the vital importance of sleep. It is our hope that this series will encourage all readers to not only obtain sufficient sleep, but to make sleep health a priority. Let's work together to enhance the value of sleep in our families and communities. If we can do this, we will all enjoy healthier, happier, more productive and safer lives.

Sweet dreams,

Terry Cralle, RN, MS
Certified Clinical Sleep Educator

W. David Brown, PhD, DABSM, CBSM
Sleep Psychologist

Recommended Amount of Sleep for Pediatric Populations: A Consensus Statement of the American Academy of Sleep Medicine

CATEGORY	AGE	NUMBER OF HOURS EACH DAY
Newborns	0–3 months	**
Infants*	4–12 months	12 to 16
Toddlers*	1–2 years	11 to 14
Preschoolers*	3–5 years	10 to 13
School-age children	6–12 years	9 to 12
Teenagers	13–18 years	8 to 10

*   Including naps.

** Recommendations for infants younger than 4 months are not included due to the wide range of normal variation in duration and patterns of sleep, and insufficient evidence for associations with health outcomes.

Paruthi S, Brooks LJ, D'Ambrosio C, Hall WA, Kotagal S, Lloyd RM, Malow BA, Maski K, Nichols C, Quan SF, Rosen CL, Troester MM, Wise MS. Recommended amount of sleep for pediatric populations: a consensus statement of the American Academy of Sleep Medicine. *J Clin Sleep Med* 2016;12(6):785–786.

I've got a secret.

When everyone is sleeping,
I'm fighting sleep!

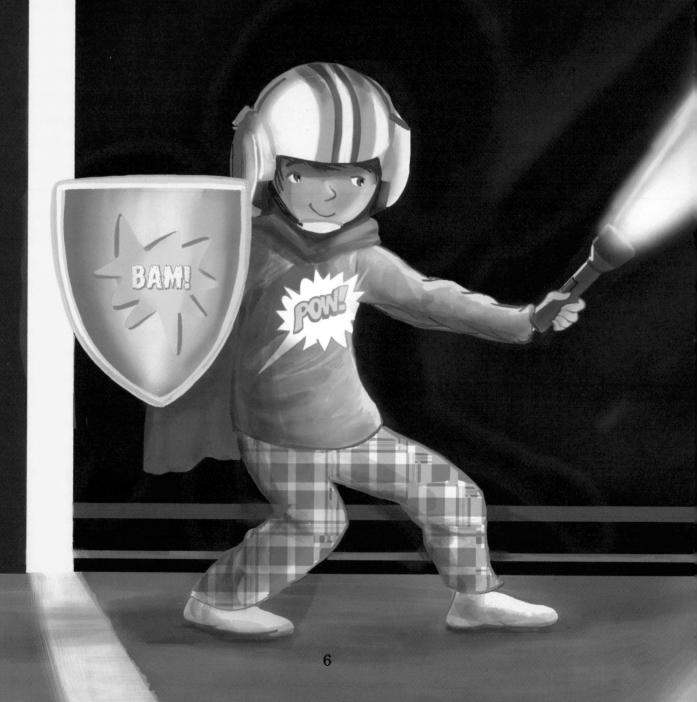

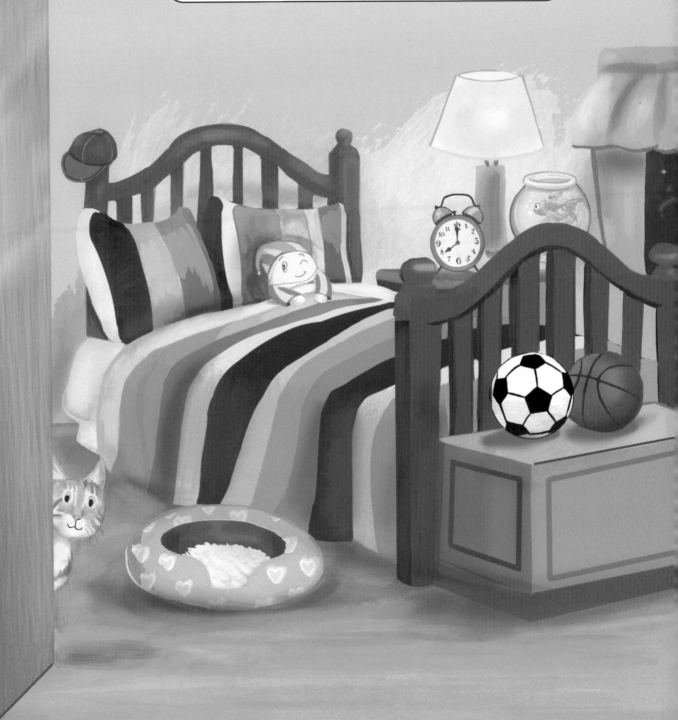

Saaaam, it's way past your bedtime — please go to sleep...

In a minute...

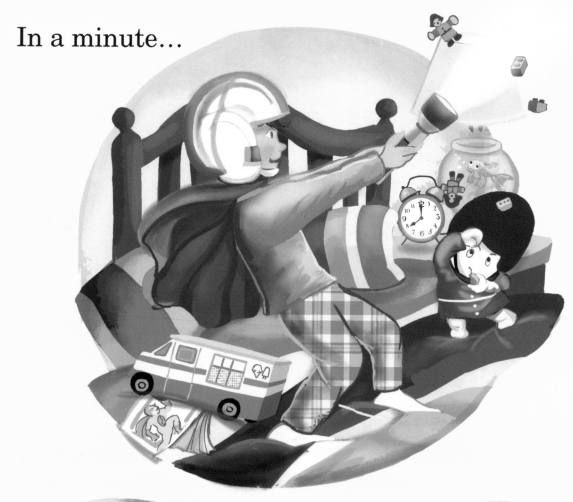

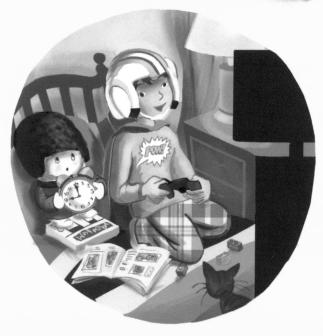

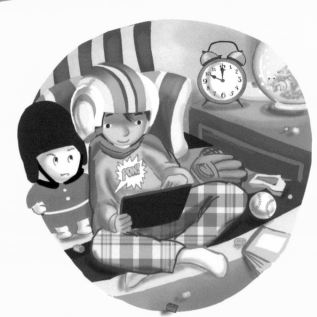

8

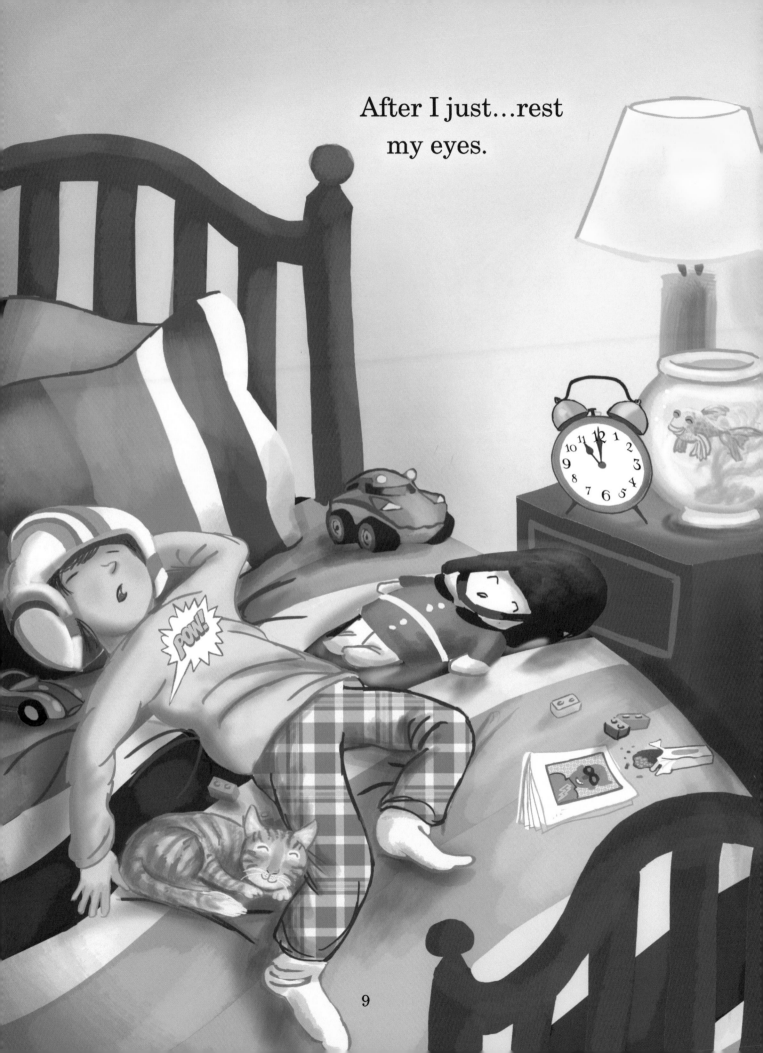

After I just...rest
my eyes.

9

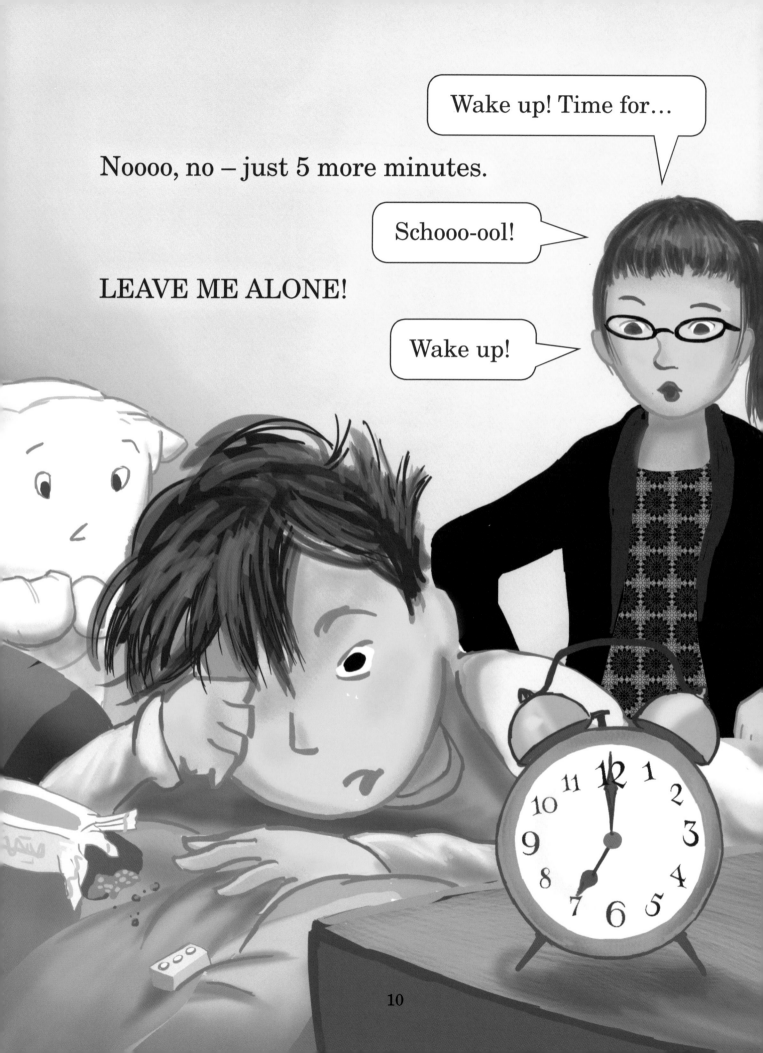

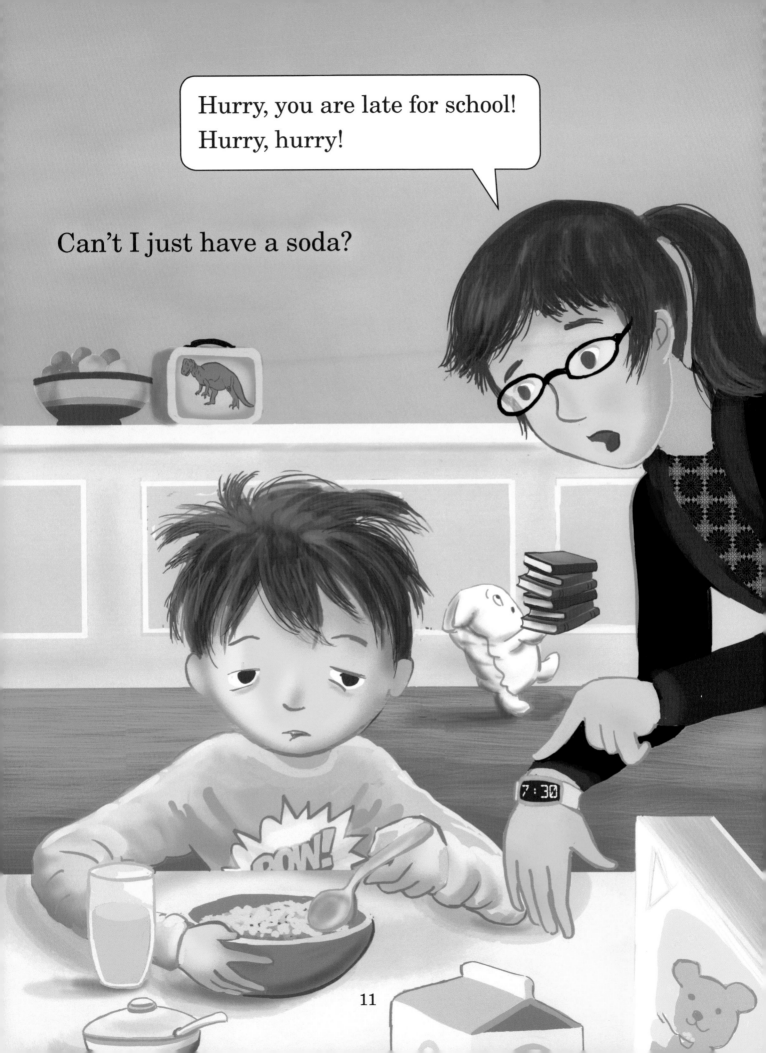

I studied that word. Why can't I remember it?

Oh, this is how you spell *sleep*:
s - l - e - e - p.

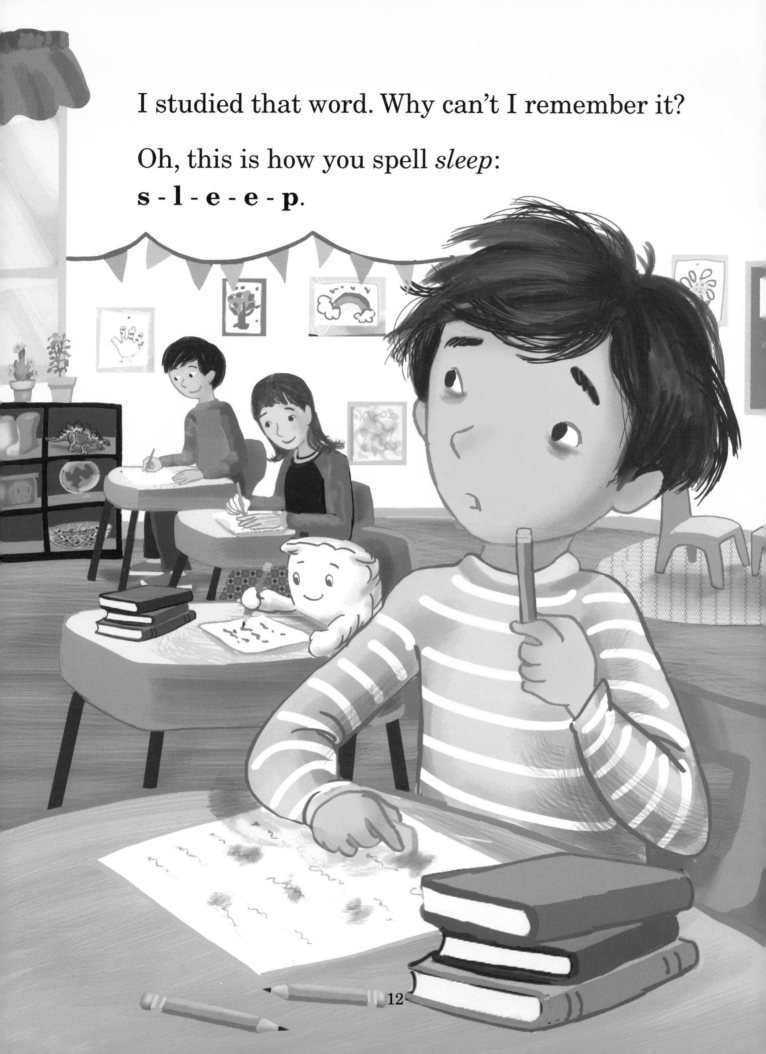

But I made that same shot six times last weekend.

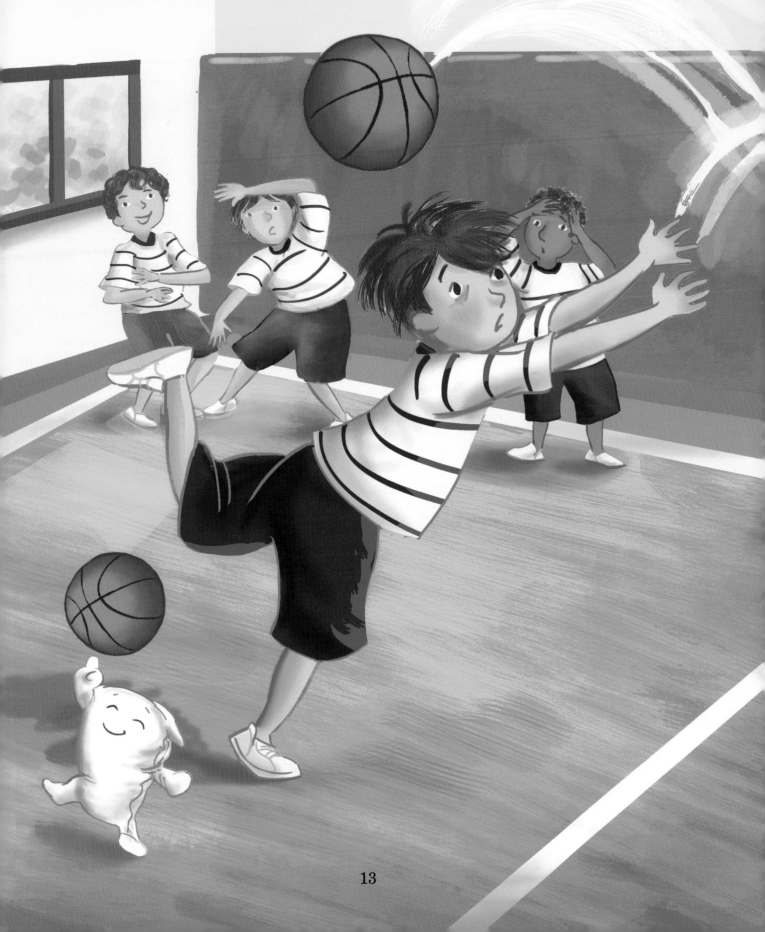

Oh no, I forgot my lunch again.

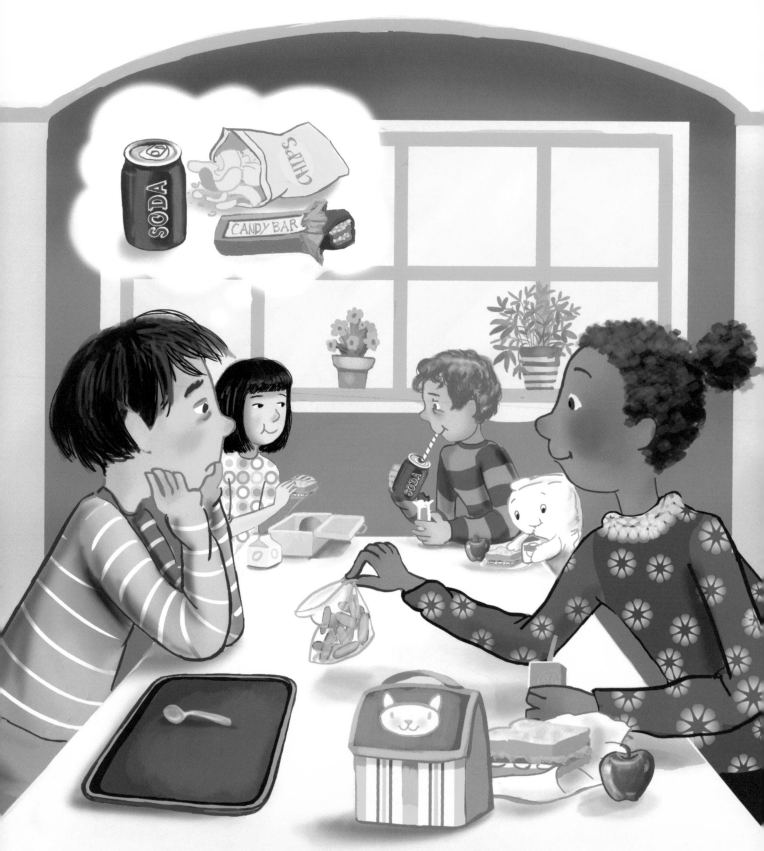

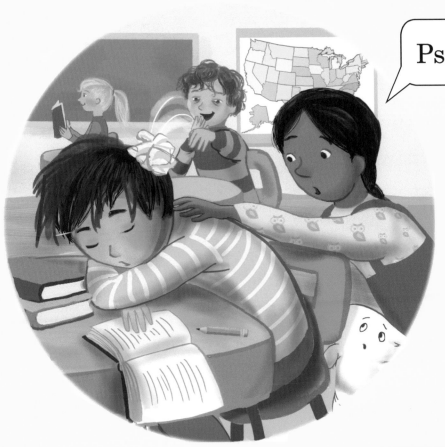

Pssssst — wake up!

It looks like
two boys are
not getting
the sleep
they need.

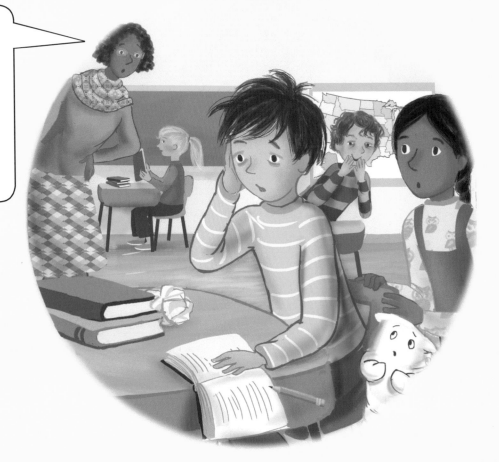

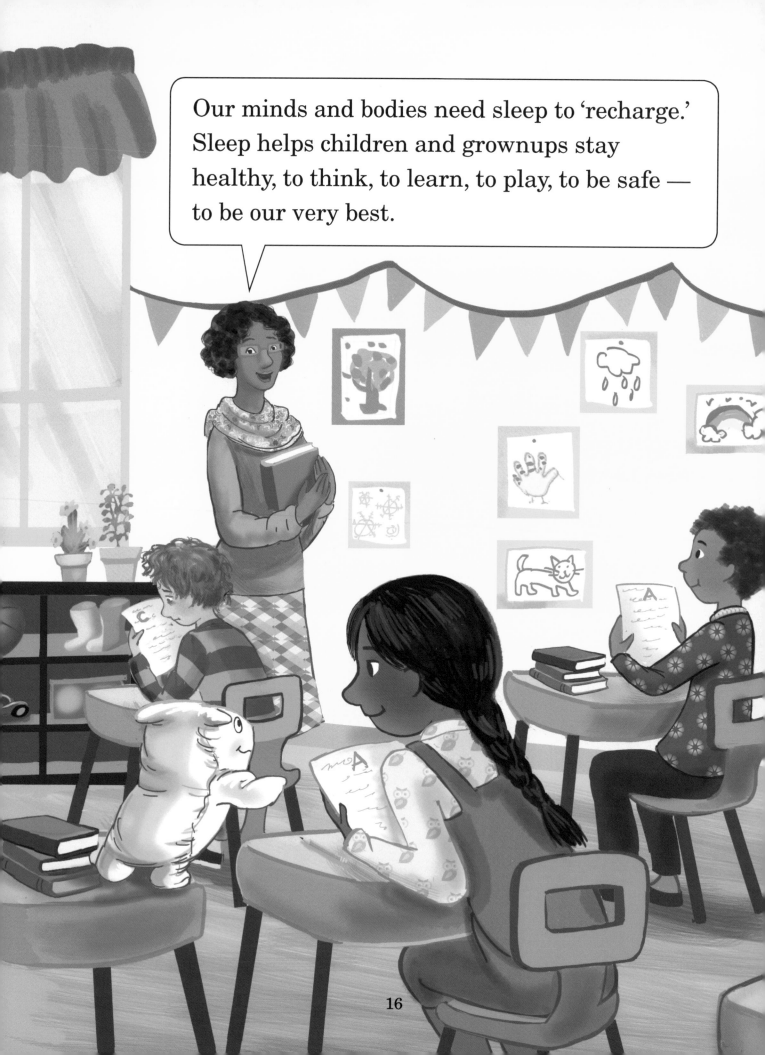

Uh-oh. I didn't do well.

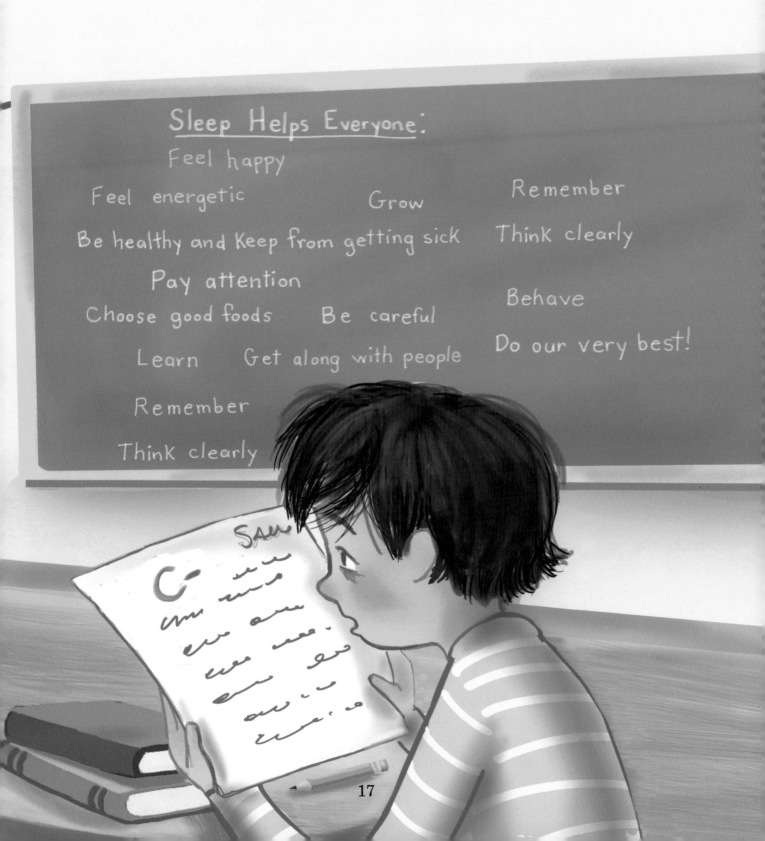

Don't fight sleep. Bedtime should not be a battle. When we get sleep:

- ☑ we **feel** better,
- ☑ we **think** better,
- ☑ we feel **happier**,
- ☑ we **play** better,
- ☑ we **eat** better,
- ☑ we **do** better, and
- ☑ we **work** better.

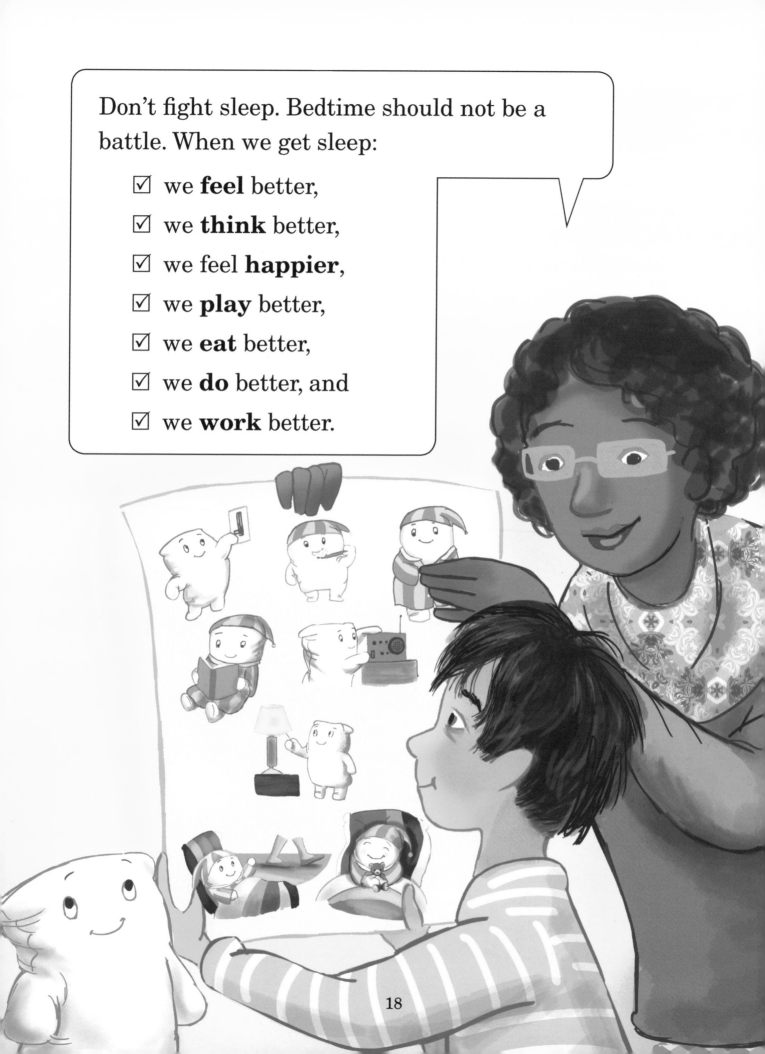

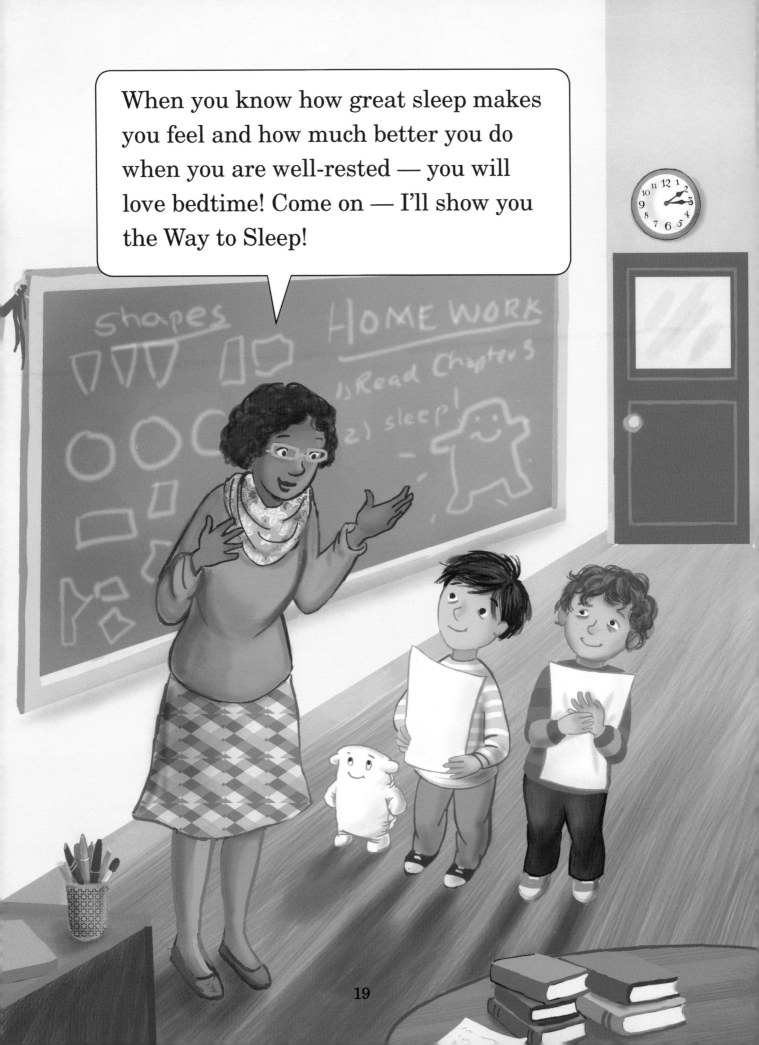

When you know how great sleep makes you feel and how much better you do when you are well-rested — you will love bedtime! Come on — I'll show you the Way to Sleep!

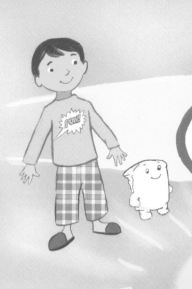

Choose a
healthy snack

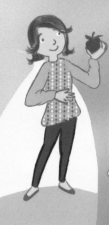

St

SNACK ATTACK!
UNHEALTHY SNACK
GO BACK 1 SPACE

HEALTHY SNACK
GO AHEAD
2 SPACES

Screens off

Dim the lights

LIGHTS ON
GO BACK
1 SPACE

BRUS
G
1

HEALTHY SNACK
GO AHEAD
2 SPACES

SNACK ATTACK!
UNHEALTHY SNACK
GO BACK 1 SPACE

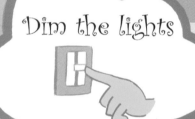

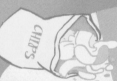

Nothing like
a warm bath

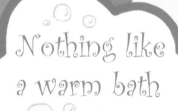

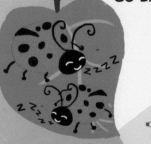

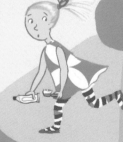

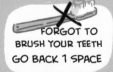

FORGOT TO
BRUSH YOUR TEETH
GO BACK 1 SPACE

Brush your teeth

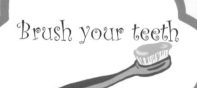

20

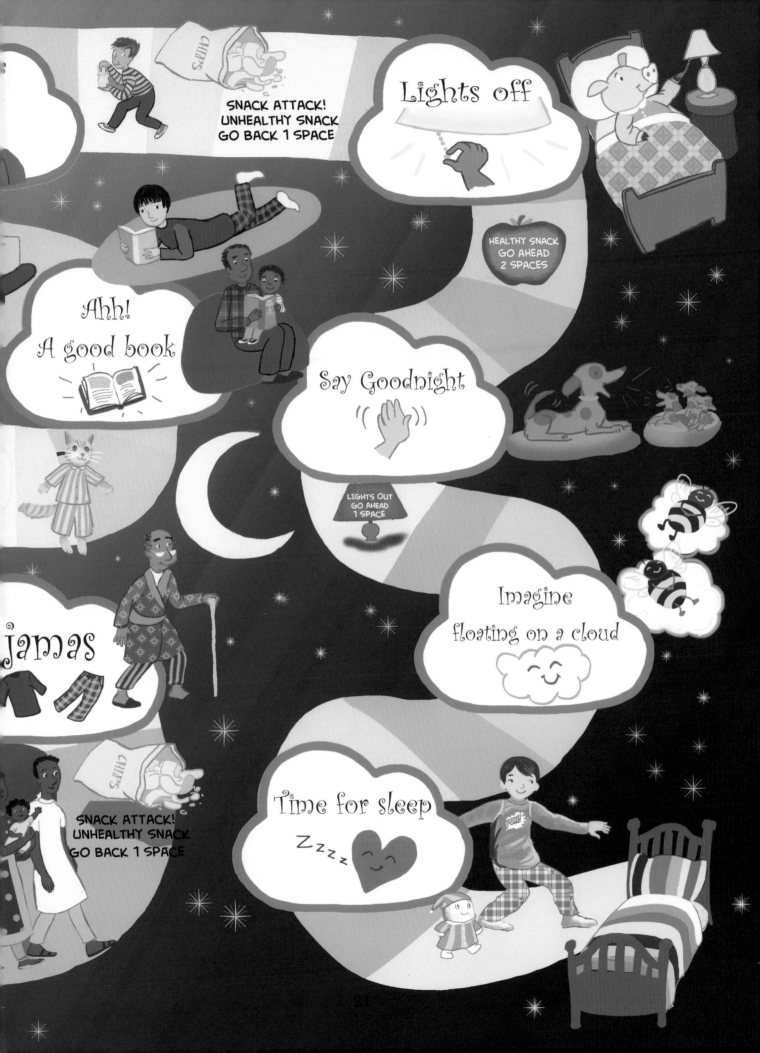

Dinner's over, homework is done.
It's time to wind down.

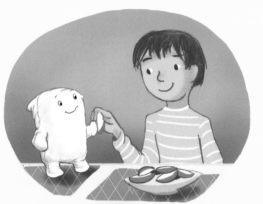

Hungry? Choose
a healthy snack.

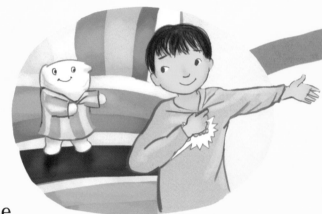

Pajamas.

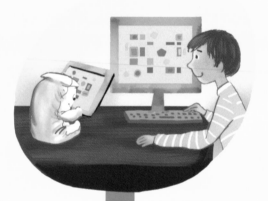

Bedtime is quiet time.
Screens off. A full hour
before bedtime.

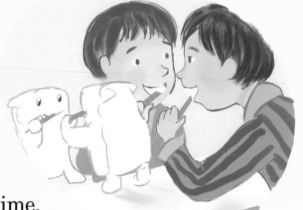

Brush your
teeth.

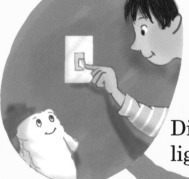

Dim the
lights.

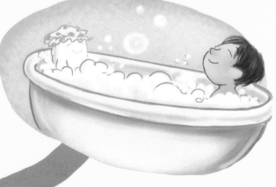

Nothing like a
warm bath.

Waking up during the night is okay. Just adjust your pillow and smile and drift back to sleep...knowing tomorrow will be a wonderful, brand new day.

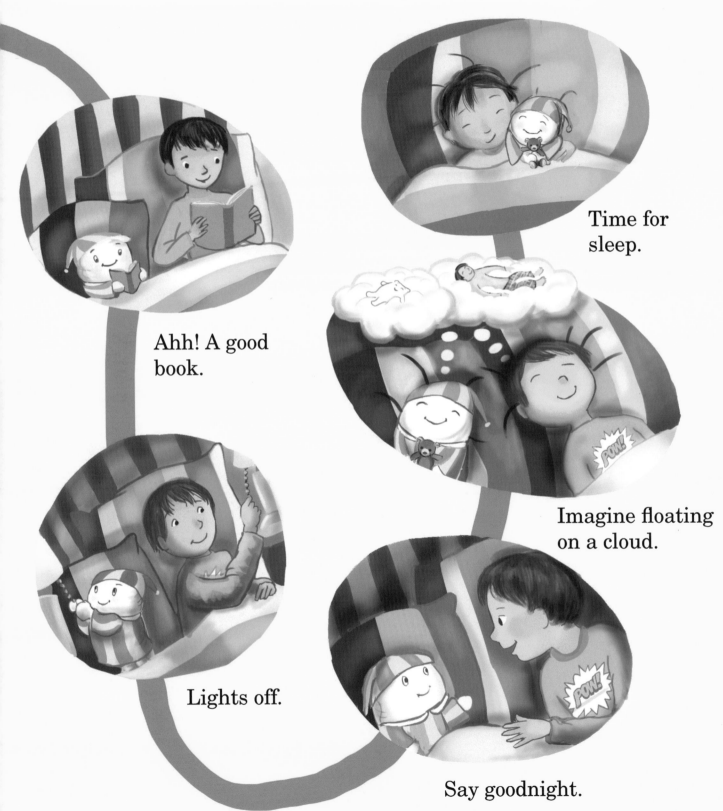

Ahh! A good book.

Time for sleep.

Imagine floating on a cloud.

Lights off.

Say goodnight.

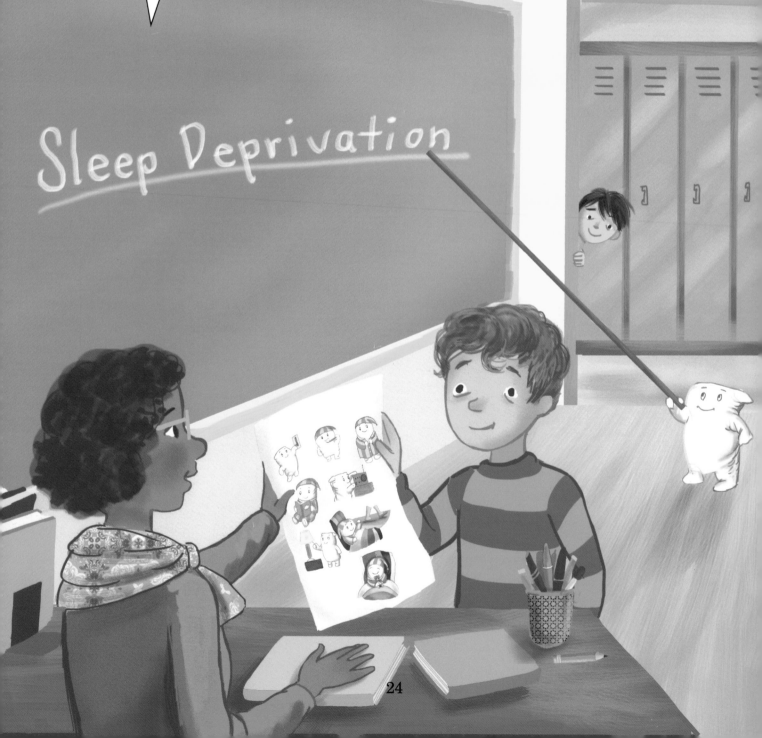

Tonight I am NOT going to fight sleep.

I will be a Sleep Superhero instead!

ZZZZZ

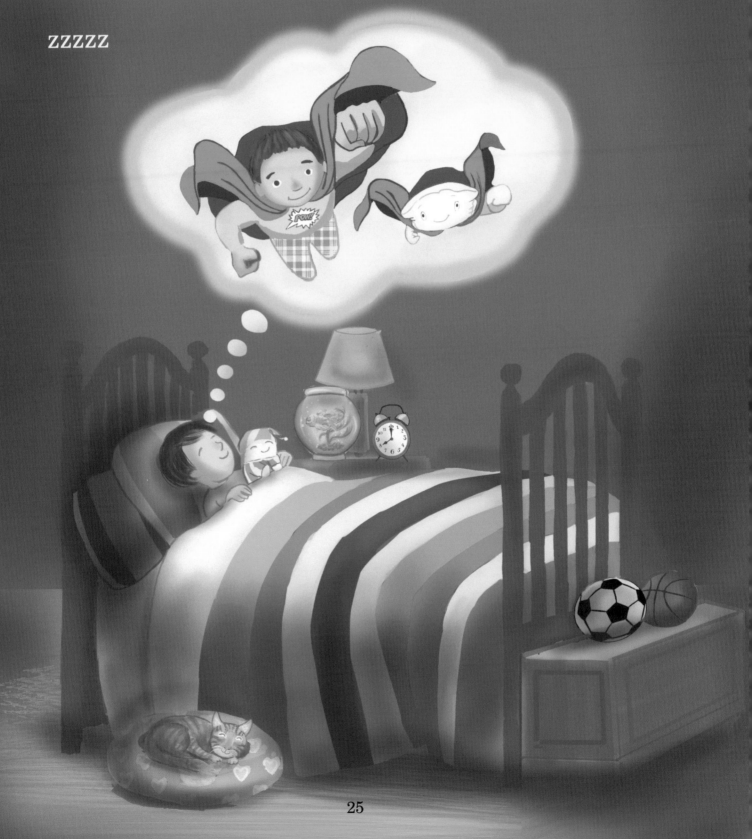

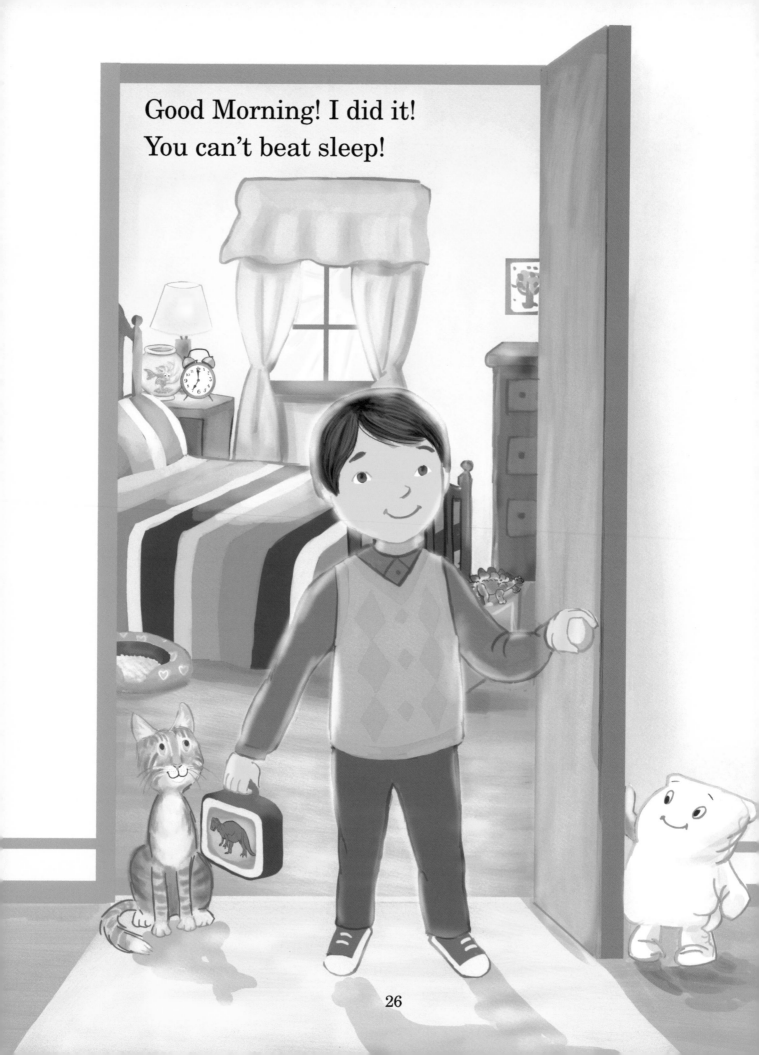

Good Morning! I did it!
You can't beat sleep!

26

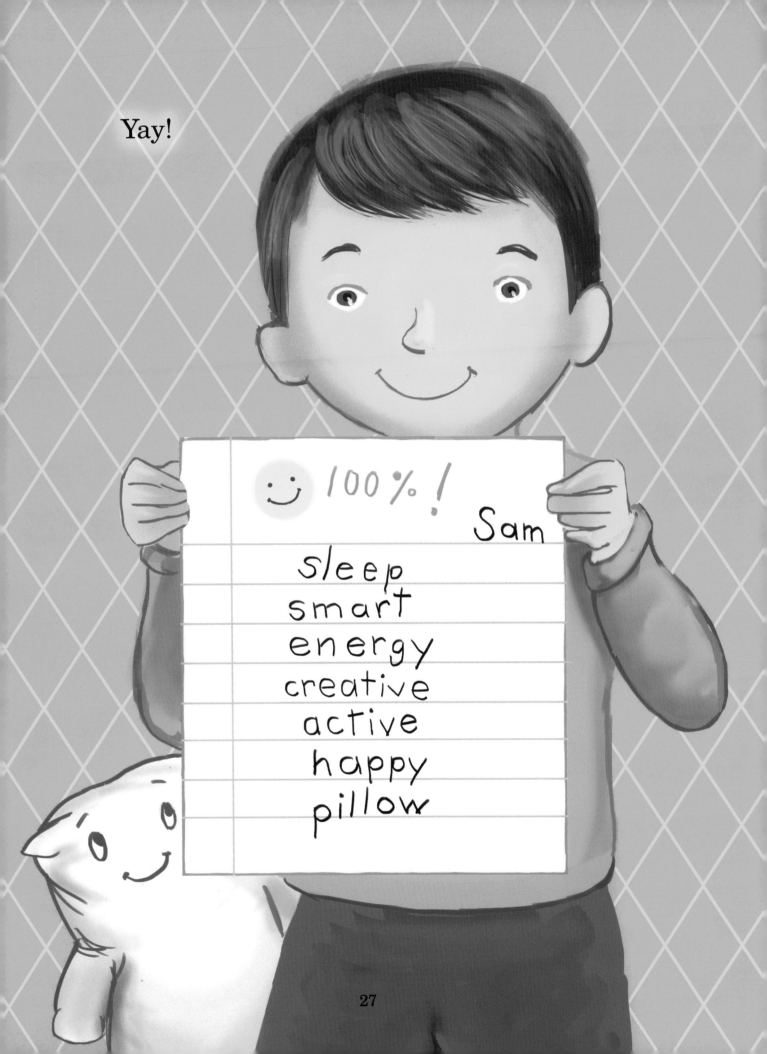

When you get sleep, you feel like a winner.

I want to win!

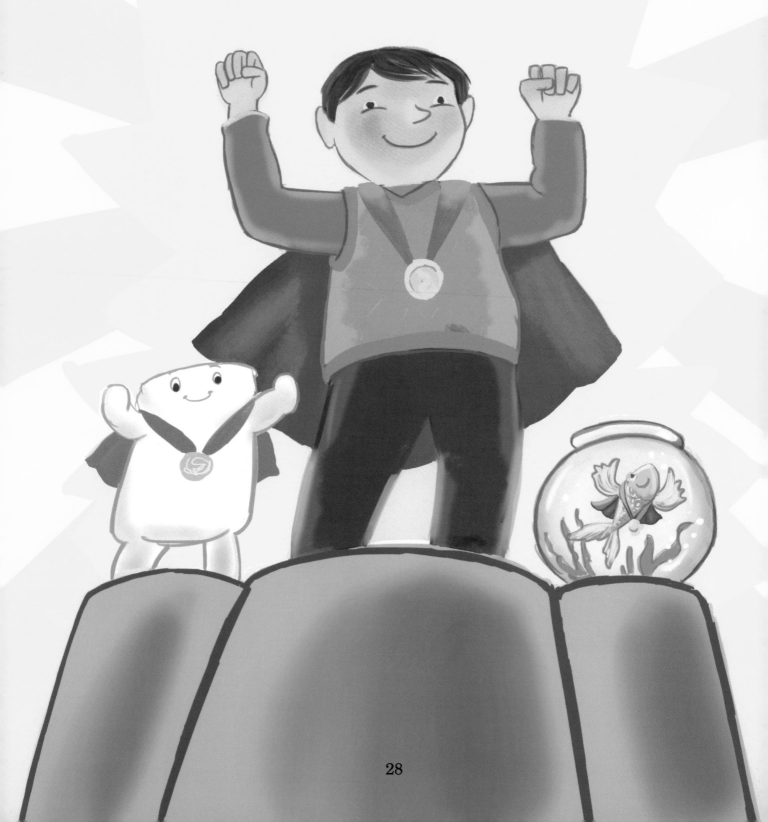

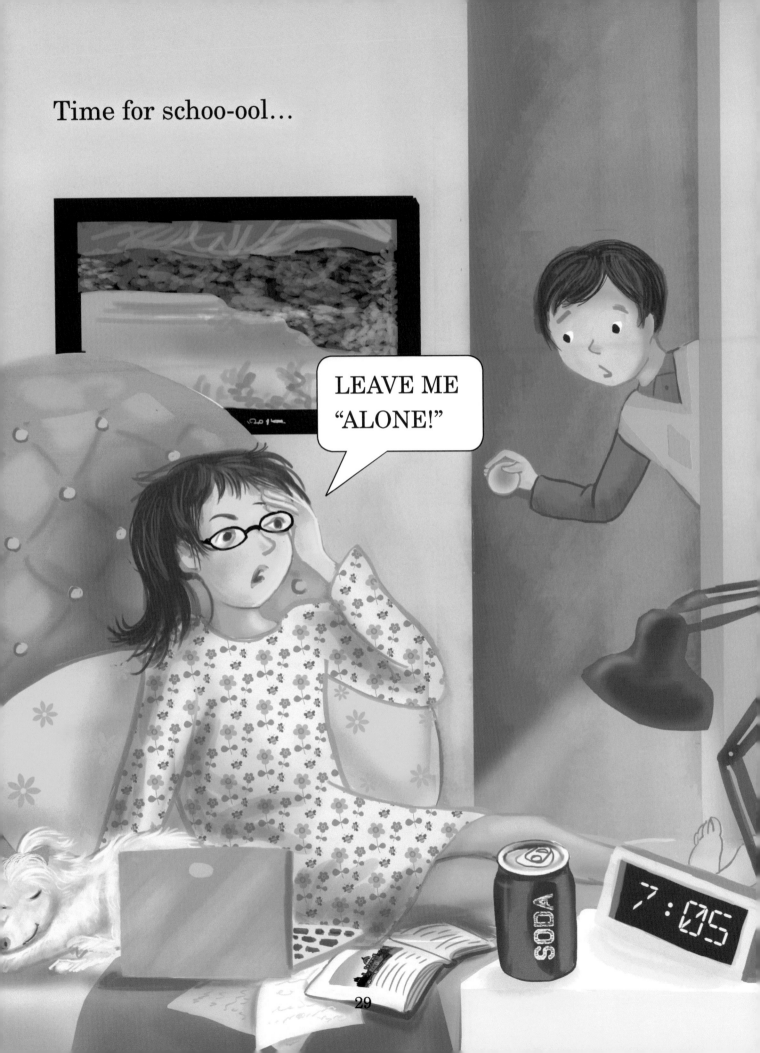

Now it's your turn to follow

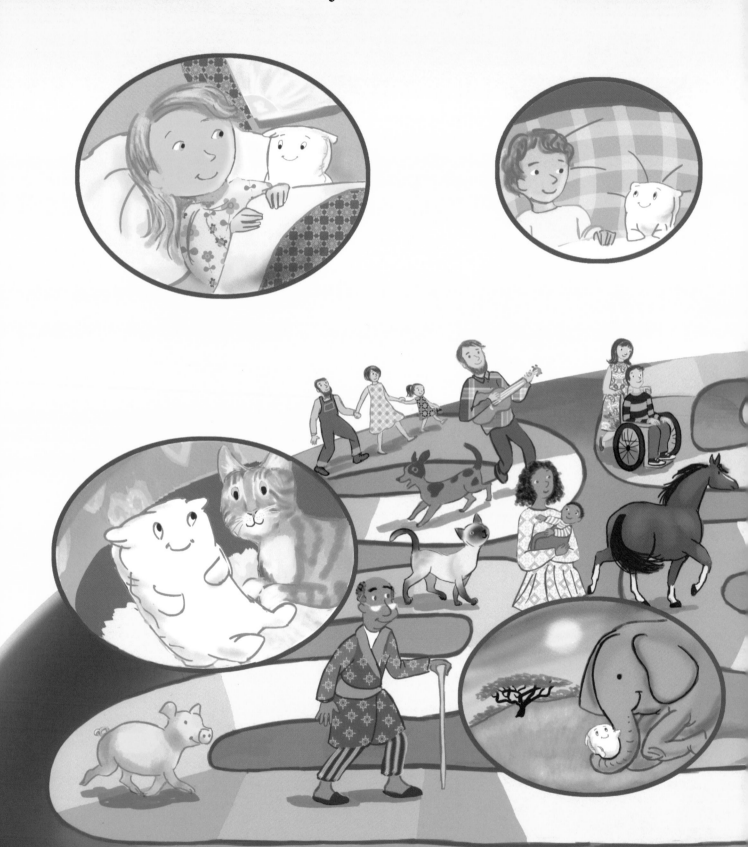

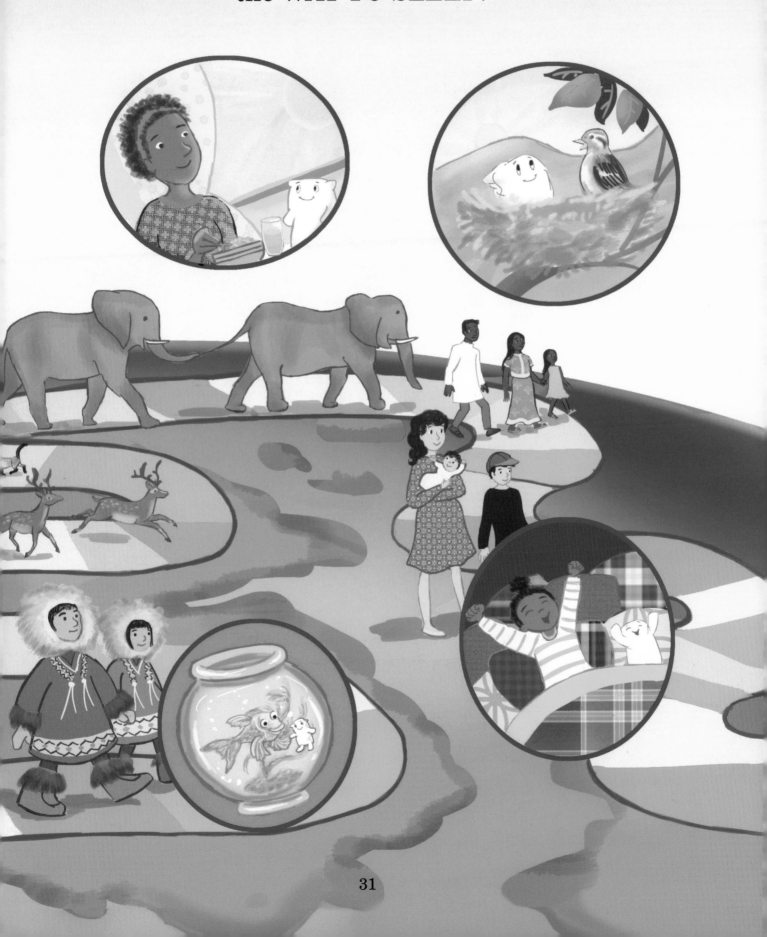

31

Let's Talk About It

Everyone needs sleep!

What animals have you seen sleeping? Do they curl up, lie down, or hang upside down? When and how long do you think they sleep? How are animals the same or different from one another when they sleep? Draw a picture of an animal sleeping.

Get a routine!

A bedtime routine is a series of things you do every night before you go to sleep. The routine should be relaxing and help you wind down and get ready to sleep. A bedtime routine helps you transition from being awake to being asleep.

What is Sam's bedtime routine? Do you have a bedtime routine that you do every night before you go to sleep? How is your bedtime routine different from Sam's? How could you improve your routine?

What time is bedtime?

Does everyone in your household have a bedtime? What time do you go to sleep at night? Draw a picture of a clock that shows your bedtime.

Add the hours between your bedtime and time that you need to wake up. Look at the chart to see if you are getting enough sleep for your age. Having a bedtime and sticking to it helps you stay healthy and happy.

Let's Talk About It

How much sleep is enough?

Do you have a hard time waking up in the morning? Or do you wake up alert and ready to go? If you feel tired in the mornings, you may not be getting the sleep you need. Some people need more sleep than others and that's OK — it's important to get the right amount of sleep that your body and mind need.

Keep a sleep diary for one week. Write down when you went to sleep. If you woke up in the middle of the night, write down what time you woke up and how you felt when you woke up. Are you getting sufficient sleep? If not, try going to bed earlier!

What details in the book tell you whether or not Sam is getting enough sleep? Do you think Sam's sister is getting enough sleep? How do you know?

How was Sam different on the day after he had a good night's sleep?

Light disturbs our sleep.

Do you avoid bright lights and electronics before bedtime? What could you do before bed that doesn't require bright light?

Sleep is important for everything we do. Sleep helps keep our bodies and minds strong and healthy. Regularly getting enough sleep helps all of us do better in school, in sports, and almost every activity of your day.

As Snoozby says, "If you feel beat, get sleep."

33

Guide to Let's Talk About It

Everyone needs sleep!

Answers will vary.

Get a routine!

Refer to pages 22-23 for Sam's routine.

What time is bedtime?

Answers will vary.

Refer to page 5 for the Sleep Requirements Based on Age.

How much sleep is enough?

Answers will vary.

Sam displayed not enough sleep by not waking up on time, too tired at breakfast, couldn't remember his school lessons, didn't perform well in gym class, forgot his lunch, falling asleep in class.

Sam's sister is not getting enough sleep either. Her light was on; she overslept; drinking soda; her computer, pet, and books were on her bed.

Sometimes misbehaving really means "I'm not getting enough sleep!" Sam's friend who threw the paper may not be getting the sleep he needs.

Light disturbs our sleep.

Answers will vary.

Things to do that does not require bright light could be puzzles, coloring, blocks, reading, and other non-electronic activities.

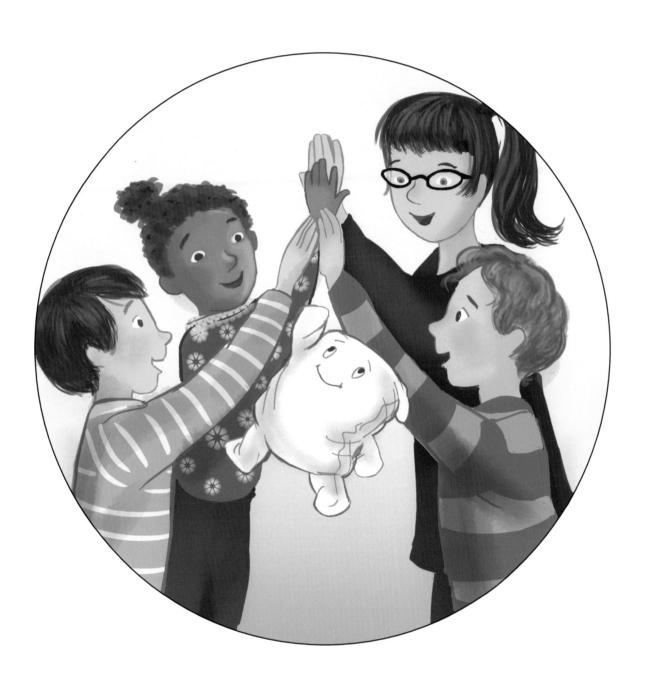

CPSIA information can be obtained at www.ICGtesting.com
Printed in the USA
BVIW12n0635300716
456848BV00004B/2